20 Surprising Foods for Clearer Vision

(with over 50 recipes!)

9/1/2015
RelaxtoClarity.com a CyberBizEnterprises, LLC Company
Dr. John DeWitt

Disclaimer:

You must not rely on the information in this book and/or video series as an alternative to medical advice from your doctor or other professional healthcare provider.

If you have any specific questions about any medical matter you should consult your doctor or other professional healthcare provider.

If you think you may be suffering from any medical condition you should seek immediate medical attention.

You should never delay seeking medical advice, disregard medical advice, or discontinue medical treatment because of information in this book and/or video series.

Any change in medication, diet, and or exercise should be directed by a qualified health care professional.

Table of Contents

Nutrition & Vision

We have always been told that nutrition is important. Some of us took that to heart and others just shrugged it off. Unfortunately those "shruggers" usually feel the costly effects later in life. In this book, I am going to reveal the foods I discovered during my quest to get clearer vision without glasses or contacts. Some may seem exotic others may seem common. The nutrients in these foods, and the over 50 recipes included, contain vital nutrients to improve vision and even heal damaged eyes.

First a little about me. I started wearing glasses in the 8th grade. I always wanted to look smart so I didn't mind. Once I started playing football in highschool, things changed. I noticed I couldn't see the ball as well as I should have. Later on in my football years, I would wear contacts during games. This proved to be extremely frustrating because I was always getting poked in the eye, getting dirt in my eyes or the worst, having a contact lens come out during a game and having to stop and look for it on my hands and knees!

I was blessed to go on to play 12 years of professional football after graduating from Vanderbilt University. My glasses and contacts, while getting more stylish in the late 80s early 90s, were still annoying.

Once I retired from football, I went on to become a Doctor of Chiropractic in Southern California. We give health talks at our office on a weekly basis so research was something I do constantly. Over two years ago I came across the work of Dr William Bates. His methods involved exercises to help the muscles of the eye to move more freely and change the shape of the eyeball itself to allow for easier focus. I was intrigued. I tried a couple of the exercises and was amazed! I found that I could see much clearer and did not wear my glasses for over two years!

I go into much more detail in my earlier book, *You Don't Need Your Glasses or Contacts.* It is available on Amazon.com.

I am a bit of a research junkie. I decided to go on an educational journey and discover everything I could about natural vision solutions. This is what lead me to discovering the specific nutrients that helped improve vision...which are found in the pages of this book.

I am a satisfied Bates student but not a Bates' practitioner. I only wish to share this information so that others who suffer with glasses, cataracts, macualr degeneration, dry eye and other debilitating conditions can get some relief. I hope you enjoy it.

Vitamin A

Remember that in order to be able to see, our specialized cells (rods and cones) located in the retina must need to function well. After the light hits these receptors they get bleached, these visual pigments need to regenerate in order to keep doing what they need to do. Vitamin A helps that regeneration process.

Vitamin C

Vitamin C strengthens the immune system to protect the body from pathogens. It has the same effect on the eyes. Vitamin C acts as an antioxidant that protects the cells in the eyes from damage caused by harmful allergens from the environment. It also promotes healing which helps maintain a healthy cornea and overall eye vitality.

Vitamin E

Vitamin E is also important for better vision. It helps in the synthesis of red blood cells which is critical for eye health. Vitamin E is most beneficial to the eyes as it can protect our visual organs from free radicals which abound in the environment.

Antioxidants

Natural antioxidants beta-carotene, zeaxanthin and lutein can also help your vision. These antioxidants may sound alien for some but these powerhouses are now commonly incorporated in all kinds of health products from bath soaps to nutritional supplements. In the eyes, they protect the macula which is located in the middle of the eye ball, from sun damage. Proper antioxidant intake helps ensure that you are taking the necessary steps to slow down age-related macular degeneration.

DHA, Omega-3s

DHA from fish oils can help strengthen your cell membranes and it can provide structural support for your eyes and boost your entire eye health. Omega 3s are also a natural anti-inflammatory and help to regenerate the cartilage of the joints. They are another nutrient that helps prevent macular degeneration.

Zinc

Zinc is a mineral that is necessary for cell division and cell division is a process necessary for healing and growth. This helps the "re-pigmentation" of the rods and cones in the retina of the eyes.

20 FOODS FOR CLEARER VISION

When you were younger, you were probably told countless times that some orange colored foods, specifically carrots, promote healthy eyes. While you may think that your parents' efforts to protect your vision were a cover up to get you to eat all your vegetables, there's some truth in what they were saying. These orange foods are more than meets the eye (no pun intended); they contain large amounts of Beta-carotene, a form of vitamin A, which is responsible for giving these orange foods their bright color. Beta-carotene is known to help restore and maintain the health of the retina, which in turn helps your eyes to function properly.

Carrots are the obvious food for better

eyesight, even our parents know this, but keeping your eyes healthy through your diet doesn't just rely on beta- carotene alone. There are a number of other beneficial vitamins and minerals that are just as important for healthy eyes.

At the end of the day, there's some truth in the old adage 'You are what you eat!' Eating healthily on a daily basis is essential for your overall health, especially your eyes' health. Here are some of the most powerful foods you should be including in your diet to help promote healthy eyes and vision.

LEAFY GREENS

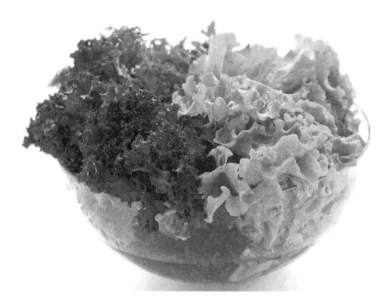

Leafy greens are also probably one of the food groups your parents were trying to get you to eat more of when you were younger, and again they're right, but probably not for the same reasons as they were advocating. Leafy greens that include kale, spinach, collard, lettuce, broccoli, and cabbage are jam-packed with a whole lot of zeaxanthin and lutein, two powerful antioxidants that have been proved to help reduce the risk of degeneration of the eye and cataracts later on in life.

SWISS CHARD SALAD WITH CRANBERRIES

Ingredients:

- 1 onion, minced

- 3 cups Swiss chard, rinsed and leaves separates

- 1 cup dried cranberries

- ¼ cup pumpkin seeds

- 1 tablespoon of grass-fed butter

- 4 cup walnuts, chopped

- ½ cup raw cane sugar

- ¼ teaspoon smoked paprika

- 2 tablespoons balsamic vinegar

- 3 tablespoons sherry vinegar

- ½ cup coconut oil

Directions:

1. In a saucepan over medium heat, melt in the grass-fed butter. Add the walnuts

and cook until lightly toasted. Remove almonds from saucepan, transfer on a plate and set aside.

2. In a mixing bowl, combine the pumpkin seeds, cane sugar, onions, balsamic vinegar, sherry vinegar, paprika and the oil. Mix it thoroughly until the sugar is completely dissolved. Set aside.

3. In a separate mixing bowl, place the Swiss chard and then pour in the liquid mixture. Gently toss to coat the chard with the dressing, stir in the cranberries and walnuts.

4. Portion salad into individual serving bowls and top with extra cranberries and walnuts. Drizzle with dressing on top and serve.

Notes

SPINACH-TOMATO HASHBROWN PIE

Ingredients:

- 1 cup soft cheese, divided

- 2 tablespoons of coconut oil

- 3 cups fresh spinach or kale leaves

- 2 to 2 ½ cups organic hash brown potatoes, thawed if frozen

- 2 garlic cloves, minced

- 1 cup of cherry tomatoes, halved

- salt and coarsely ground black pepper, to taste

- 3 organic eggs

- ¼ cup coconut milk

- pinch of ground nutmeg

Directions:

1. Preheat oven to 375°F.

2. Lightly grease a 9-inch pie plate with oil, add and press down the hash brown potatoes into the pie plate.

3. Bake it in the oven for about 8 minutes, or until lightly brown. Remove from the oven and top off with half of the soft cheese, set aside.

4. In a pan over medium heat, melt in the coconut oil. Stir in the spinach and tomatoes, cook for 3 to 4 minutes or until spinach is wilted, stirring frequently. Stir in the garlic and continue to cook for another 1 minute. Remove from heat and add it on top of the baked potatoes.

5. In a mixing bowl, whisk together the coconut milk, eggs, nutmeg and season to taste with salt and pepper. Thoroughly whisk the ingredients until the salt is completely dissolved.

6. Pour over the egg-milk mixture over the wilted spinach. Top with the remaining cheese and bake it in the oven for 30 to 35 minutes. When the top part turns golden brown, it is done.

7. Remove from the oven and let it stand for at least 10 minutes. Slice then serve.

Notes

KALE STRAWBERRY BANANA SMOOTHIE

Ingredients:

- 1 tablespoon chia seeds

- ½ pound strawberries, frozen

- ½ cup of water

- 1 ½ tablespoons organic lemon juice

- 2 cups baby kale, roughly chopped

- 1 ripe banana, chopped

Directions:

1. In blender, add and combine the strawberries, chia seeds, lemon juice, kale and the banana. Pulse ingredients to coarse mixture then add the water. Pulse again until a smooth and frothy.

2. Transfer smoothie into individual serving glasses, serve immediately.

Notes

EGGS

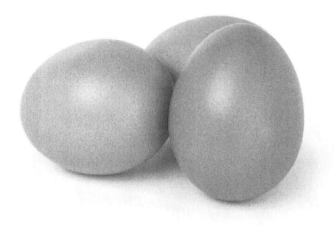

It doesn't matter if they're boiled, scrambled, fried or in an omelet, eggs are an excellent source of nutrition for your eyes. The yolk of the egg is especially powerful as it contains a good amount of lutein, zeaxanthin, and zinc. Like your leafy greens, the egg yolk can help maintain your eyes' health as you grow older, and essentially it can help fight cataracts. The yolk of an egg also contains a great source of natural vitamin D, which over the years has been proved to help reduce the risk of developing ARMD (age-related macular degeneration), which results in vision loss later on in life.

Notes

ASPARAGUS AND EGG PIZZA

Ingredients:

- 1 pound gluten-free pizza dough, divided into 2 balls

- 1 cup semi-soft cheese, grated

- 1 pound asparagus, trimmed and cut into bias

- 1/2 small yellow onion, thinly sliced crosswise

- 1 1/2 tablespoons coconut oil

- salt and ground black pepper, to taste

- 2 stems of chives, finely chopped

- Coconut flour for dusting

- 4 large organic eggs

- ½ cup Parmesan cheese, grated

Directions:

1. Preheat an oven to 500°F. Lightly grease 2 baking sheets and set aside.

2. Ina large mixing bowl, add and combine the asparagus, the onion, oil and season to taste with salt and pepper.

3. Lightly flour a work surface, bring the dough balls over the work surface. Roll out the doughs into 10-inch rounds with a rolling pin, transfer into the greased baking sheet.

4. Top the round doughs with cheese and asparagus and bake it in the oven for about 10 minutes. Once the edges are slightly charred and the asparagus starts to soften, remove from the oven and crack 2 eggs on each. Return in the oven and bake for about 3 to 4 minutes or until the egg whites are cooked but the yellows are still runny.

5. Transfer the pizzas to a cutting board, and sprinkle with the Parmigiano-

Reggiano and chives. Slice and serve, making sure everyone gets some egg.

Notes

EASY EGG CUSTARD

Ingredients:

- 2 egg yellows from organic eggs
- 4 tablespoons raw cane sugar
- 2 cups coconut milk
- 2 organic eggs
- ½ tablespoon almonds extract
- A pinch of nutmeg

Directions:

1. Preheat an oven to a temperature of 300°F. Place the custard cups in a deep baking pan and set aside.

2. In a mixing bowl, whisk together the eggs, sugar, and almond extract until the sugar is completely dissolved.

3. Add the coconut milk in a saucepan and apply with medium heat. When the milk is hot, pour in the egg mixture and slowly whisk until the ingredients are

well combined. Stir in the nutmeg then remove from heat.

4. Pour mixture into the custard cups and add warm water in the baking pan just enough to cover the cups in half.

5. Bake it in the oven for 30 to 35 minutes. Remove from the oven and transfer custard cups in baking pan with water bath, cool for 2 hours before serving.

Notes

AVOCADO DEVILED EGGS

Ingredients:

- 1 organic lime, juiced

- 1/2 cup Greek yogurt

- 10 organic eggs, boiled and shelled

- 1/2 medium avocado, pitted and diced

- 1/2 teaspoon salt

- Fresh cilantro, for garnish

Directions:

1. Cut eggs in half crosswise. Take out the yolks and place it in a mixing bowl, place the whites on a plate and set aside.

2. In a mixing bowl with the yolks, mix in the avocado, yogurt, lime juice and salt. Mix to combine.

3. Place mixture in piping bag and pipe into the egg whites. Top eggs with chopped cilantro then serve.

Notes

LEMON

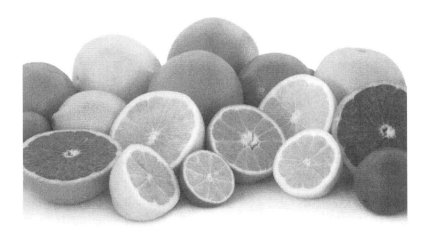

Oranges, lemons, limes, and grapefruit are all full of vitamin C. Vitamin C is superior to most other vitamins, and it's one of the best forms of antioxidants. Vitamin C is known to form and maintain your body's connective tissues, which also includes the collagen found in your eye's cornea. Eating more citrus fruit will help protect your eyes from trauma to the eyes and prevent them from being damaged.

LEMON MERINGUE

Ingredients:

- 4 organic egg yolks, beaten

- 4 organic egg whites

- 1 cup raw cane sugar

- 1 packet stevia

- 2 tablespoons almond flour

- 3 tablespoons arrowroot flour

- 2 tablespoons grass-fed butter

- 1/4 teaspoon salt

- 1 1/2 cups water

- 2 organic lemons, juiced and zested

- 1 pie crust (9-inch), baked ahead

Directions:

1. Preheat an oven to a temperature of 350°F.

2. In a mixing bowl, mix together the 1 cup sugar, flour, and salt until evenly

distributed. Mix in the water, lemon juice and zest. Transfer mixture into a sauce pan and apply medium-high heat, bring the mixture to a boil while stirring occasionally and stir in the butter.

3. In a separate bowl, whisk the egg yolks thoroughly and then gradually whisk in ½ cup of hot sugar mixture. Pour yolk-sugar mixture in the saucepan, cook until thick while stirring constantly. Return to a boil and then remove saucepan from heat, pour into the baked pie crust. Set aside.

4. In a glass mixing bowl, whisk the egg whites until thick and foamy. Gradually add in the stevia and continue to whisk until soft peak forms. Add meringue in the pie, spread evenly with a spatula and completely cover to seal the edges.

5. Bake it in the oven for about 10 to 12 minutes, or until golden brown. Remove from the oven and let it stand for 5 minutes before serving.

Notes

SPICY GARLIC-LIME CHICKEN

Ingredients:

- 2 to 3 tablespoons grass-fed butter

- Ground black pepper, to taste

- 1 tablespoon coconut oil

- 1/2 teaspoon crushed red chili pepper flakes

- 1 tablespoon mixed Italian herbs

- ¼ teaspoon of Pimenton (sweet smoked paprika)

- 4 organic chicken breast fillets

- 1/8 teaspoon onion salt

- 2 organic limes, juiced

- 1/4 teaspoon garlic salt

- 2 teaspoons garlic powder

Directions:

1. Combine together cayenne, mixed Italian herbs, Pimenton, crushed red

pepper flakes, garlic salt, onion salt and ground pepper in a mixing bowl. Rub the chicken evenly with the spice mixture and make sure to apply on all areas.

2. Place a skillet on the stove, apply medium heat and melt in the butter. Once the butter has melted, fry the breast fillets for about 5 to 7 minutes or until golden brown. Flip it over and cook the other side for about 5 to 6 minutes, or until lightly brown. Stir in the lemon juice and garlic powder, stir and baste with the sauce. Cover with lid and cook for 5 minutes more.

3. Remove from heat and transfer into a serving platter or individual serving plates. Drizzle with cooking sauce on top, serve with extra Italian herbs on top.

Notes

MANDARIN SALAD

Ingredients:

- 1/2 cup walnuts, chopped

- 2 tablespoons of local honey

- 1 purple onion, sliced into thin rings

- 1 cup canned mandarin oranges, drained

- 4 cups dark lettuce leaves, torn or leaves separated

- 1 cups of dried cranberries, chopped

- 1 cup Feta cheese, crumbled

- Salt and pepper, to taste

- 1 cup homemade salad dressing or vinaigrette, or as needed to taste

Directions:

1. In a mixing bowl, mix together the oranges, walnuts, cheese, onions and cranberries. Stir in the honey and gently toss the ingredients to coat. Season to taste with salt and pepper. Set aside.

2. Portion dark lettuce into individual serving bowls or platter. Top with mixed ingredients and drizzle with vinaigrette, serve with extra cheese on top.

Notes

SEEDS AND NUTS

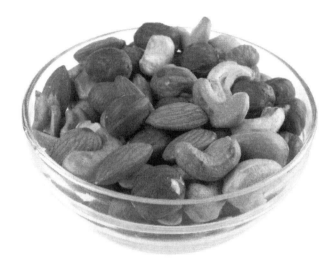

Seeds and nuts may be your favorite snack food, but they're also more beneficial than this, they're excellent sources of vitamins C and E. When combined, these vitamins work together to help keep your body's tissues strong and healthy which is essential for healthy eyes as the dense outer layer of the eye is made up of tissues. Eat more sunflower seeds, chia seeds, flaxseeds, almonds, peanuts, and pecans.

THAI COCONUT PUMPKIN SOUP

Ingredients:

- 2 cups pumpkin, peeled and diced
- 1 tablespoon coconut oil
- 1 tablespoon grass-fed butter
- ¼ cup of fresh basil leaves, chopped
- 1 teaspoon of minced garlic
- 4 shallots, diced
- 2 small fresh red hot chili, chopped
- 1 tablespoon chopped lemongrass (white part only)
- 2 cups organic chicken broth
- 1 cup coconut milk

Directions:

1. In a saucepan over medium-low heat, add the oil and butter. Once the butter has melted, sauté in the chili, chopped lemongrass, garlic and shallots until soft and fragrant. Pour in the organic

chicken broth coconut milk and diced pumpkin. Bring to a boil, reduce to low heat and simmer for 10 minutes or until the pumpkin is cooked through. Remove saucepan from heat, let it rest to cool.

2. When the mixture has lowered in temperature, place it in a blender and pulse mixture until you have a smooth and thick consistency. Return soup in the saucepan, reheat for about 5 minutes.

3. Portion soup into individual serving bowls, serve with fresh basil leaves on top.

Notes

TRAIL MIX HONEY POWER BARS

Ingredients:

- 1 ½ cup of organic trail mix

- 1/4 cup nut or grass-fed butter

- ½ cup quick cooking oats

- 1/4 cup raw cane sugar or 1 tablespoon of stevia powder

- ½ cup whole-grain cereal, puffed

- A pinch of salt

- 1/4 cup honey

- 1/2 teaspoon almond extract

- Coconut oil, for greasing

Directions:

1. Preheat oven to 350°F.

2. Place the oats and organic trail mix in a rimmed baking sheet and bake for about 10 minutes or until the ingredients are lightly toasted. Remove from the oven

and transfer into a bowl, stir in the cereals and toss to combine.

3. In a pan over medium-low heat, combine together the butter, honey, almond extract and salt. Cook for about 4 to 5 minutes while stirring the ingredients occasionally.

4. Combine the toasted ingredients and the how liquid mixture and transfer into a covered container, pressing down with hands to make a firm layer. Let it rest to lower in temperature.

5. Freeze for at least 30 minutes, remove from the fridge and cut into bars.

Notes

CITRUS SALAD WITH TOASTED SEEDS AND PINE NUTS

Ingredients:

- 1 small red grapefruit, peeled and segmented

- ½ cup organic mixed seeds, toasted

- 1 shallot, minced

- 1 navel orange, peeled and segmented

- 2 teaspoons of local honey

- 1 teaspoon Dijon mustard

- ½ organic lemon, juiced

- 2 tablespoons white wine vinegar

- 1/3 cup coconut oil

- Salt and freshly ground black pepper

- 2 heads Romaine lettuce, rinsed and drained, torn

- 1 cup fresh tarragon, leaves separated and roughly chopped

Directions:

1. In a pan over medium heat, add the mixed seeds and toast for about 5 to 7 minutes or until lightly toasted and fragrant. Remove pan from heat, set aside.

2. In a mixing bowl, combine together the mustard, lemon juice, vinegar and honey. Stir to combine and whisk in the coconut oil, season to taste with salt and pepper.

3. Mix in the lettuce leaves, tarragon, orange and grapefruit in separate bowl. Add the dressing and toasted seeds, and then gently toss to coat salad ingredients with the dressing.

4. Portion lettuce into individual serving bowls or plates, drizzle with dressing and top with nuts and serve.

Notes

BLUEBERRIES

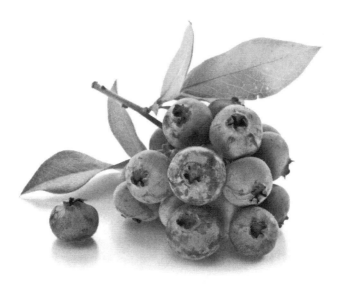

If there was a super fruit, it would surely be the blueberry. It is unbelievable how one little fruit can contain so much goodness. This humble berry is in fact one of the foods with the highest amounts of antioxidants. While the blueberry is beneficial in many ways and tackles a number of health concerns, it's especially beneficial when it comes to maintaining your eyes' health.

Blueberries contain high doses of vitamin C,

which help fight the free radicals responsible for damaging your eyes and causing eye disease. Getting more vitamin C in your diet will help reduce any intraocular pressure on the eye, meaning you'll have less of a chance of developing glaucoma later on in life, which is the second leading cause of blindness in adults in the US.

BLUEBERRY-CREAM CHEESE HAND PIES

Ingredients:

- 3/4 cup raw cane sugar

- 1 organic lemon, juiced and zested

- 1 to 2 tablespoons of cream

- 1 ½ packet stevia

- 1 organic egg

- 1 ½ cup frozen blueberries

- 1 cup cream cheese

- 2 tablespoons almond flour

- 4 to 6 gluten-free pie dough

Directions:

1. Preheat an oven to a temperature of 400°F.

2. In a mixing bowl, mix together the cheese, ½ cup cane sugar, lemon zest. Whisk the ingredients until smooth.

3. In a separate bowl, add blueberries with the remaining sugar, lemon zest, flour and egg. Toss to coat the blueberries evenly.

4. Roll out the dough into thin rounds; place it on a lined baking sheet with parchment paper. Add a tablespoon of cream cheese mixture on the center, and then top with 2 tablespoons of coated blueberries. Lightly brush the dough edges with cream, fold the edges and trim excess dough to form triangles. Crimp the edges or press down with a fork to seal, lightly brush with cream on top and dust with stevia on top. Repeat the procedure with the remaining dough.

5. Bake it in the oven for about 20 to 25 minutes, or until the dough is browned. Remove from the oven and let it stand

for about 5 minutes on a wire rack before serving.

Notes

FLANK STEAK WITH BLUEBERRY SAUCE

Ingredients:

- 1 kg grass-fed beef flank steak

- 2 garlic cloves, minced

- 1 shallot, minced

- 1 cup of fresh blueberries

- 1 cup organic beef stock

- salt and coarsely ground black pepper

- ⅓ cup red wine

- 1 teaspoon fresh thyme leaves, minced

- 2 to 3 tablespoons of ghee/clarified butter

Directions:

1. Mix the salt and pepper in a bowl. Season flank steak with generous amounts of salt-pepper mixture. Set aside.

2. In a pan over medium heat, add in the clarified butter. Once the butter is hot, sauté in the garlic and shallots until soft and fragrant. Pour in the red wine, stock and thyme and bring to a boil. Reduce to low heat and simmer for 10 minutes.

3. Transfer into a preheated skillet with 1 tablespoon of ghee and sear for about 4 to 5 minutes on each side. Pour in the cooking sauce from the pan and cook for another 3 to 4 minutes.

4. Stir in the blueberries, adjust the seasoning and cook for 2 minutes. Remove the steak and blueberries, transfer into a plate. Set aside.

5. Continue to cook the sauce with low heat until it has reduced into half. Pour sauce on top of the steak and serve.

Notes

BLUEBERRY WALNUT SALAD RECIPE

Ingredients:

- 2 cups of fresh blueberries

- 1/4 cup walnuts, chopped

- 2 cups kale or mixed salad greens

- 1/2 cup raspberry vinaigrette dressing

- 1/4 cup goat's cheese, crumbled

Directions:

1. In a mixing bowl, mix in the kale or salad greens with blueberries and chopped walnuts.

2. Pour over the raspberry vinaigrette dressing and gently toss to coat. Portion greens into individual serving bowls and top with crumbled cheese on top. Serve immediately.

Notes

SWEET POTATOES

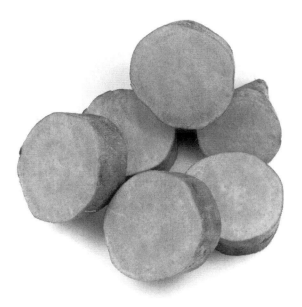

If you're not already substituting potatoes for sweet potatoes, this may make you think again. Sweet potatoes aren't only for Thanksgiving; this delicious and understated vegetable is packed with vitamin A, a powerful antioxidant. Vitamin A is responsible for protecting your eyes against any nasty free radicals that can harm your eyes. Vitamin A is particularly helpful by reducing eye inflammation and dry eyes, which are two things that if left untreated, could lead to some more serious eye problems later on down the road.

CREAMY CHICKEN CURRY WITH SWEET POTATO

Ingredients:

- ½ cup canned peas, drained

- 2 organic chicken breast fillets, cut into cubes

- 2 medium sweet potatoes, peeled and cubed

- 1 tablespoon coconut oil

- 2 teaspoons curry paste

- 4 tablespoons red split lentils

- 1 cup of organic chicken broth

- 1 ½ cups coconut milk

Directions:

1. In a deep wok or frying pan over medium-high heat, add in the oil. Once the oil is hot, add the curry paste and cook for 1 minute while stirring constantly. Stir in the chicken pieces,

cubed potatoes and lentils. Cook for 5 minutes while stirring occasionally and then pour in the stock and coconut milk. Bring to a boil, reduce to low heat and simmer for 15 minutes.

2. Add the peas and return to a boil. Cover with lid and simmer for another 5 minutes, season to taste with salt and pepper.

3. Once the vegetables are soft and cooked through, remove from heat and transfer into individual serving bowls. Serve warm.

Notes

SHEPHERD'S VEGETABLE PIE WITH MASHED SWEET POTATO

Ingredients:

- 2 cups of canned stewed tomatoes

- ½ kg of sweet potatoes, peeled and cubed

- 1 tablespoon coconut oil

- 1 medium onion, halved thinly sliced

- 2 medium carrots, peeled and cubed

- ¼ cup fresh thyme leaves, chopped

- ½ cup red wine

- ½ organic vegetable broth

- 2 cups canned green lentils

- 2 tablespoons grass-fed butter

- ¼ cup Parmesan cheese, grated

Directions:

1. In a pan over medium heat, add in the oil. Once the oil is hot, add the carrots,

stewed tomatoes, onions and half the thyme. Cook for 5 minutes while stirring occasionally. Pour in the broth and red wine and bring to a boil. Add the lentils and reduce to low heat, simmer for 10 minutes or until the vegetables are half cooked.

2. In a pot with boiling water, boil the potatoes and cooked until soft. Drain and mash with butter, season to taste with salt and pepper. Set aside.

3. Place the cooked vegetables into a greased baking dish and add cover with the mashed potatoes. Top with cheese and the remaining thyme. Chill the pie before cooking.

4. Preheat the oven to 400°F. Bake the pie for about 40 minutes if chilled and 20 minutes if not, or until the top is golden and the filling is cooked through.

Remove from the oven and transfer into a wire rack, let it stand for 5 minutes before serving.

Notes

WALNUT-MAPLE WITH SWEET POTATOES

Ingredients

- 2 tablespoons chopped walnuts

- 1/4 cup cream

- 3 tablespoons grass-fed butter, melted

- 2 to 3 tablespoons maple syrup

- 1 kg of sweet potatoes

- 1 teaspoon salt

- ½ teaspoon freshly ground black pepper

- ¼ teaspoon almond extract

- ¼ teaspoon cinnamon

- ¼ teaspoon allspice mix

- 1 large organic egg, beaten

- Oil, for greasing

Directions:

1. Preheat an oven to a temperature of 400°F. Line a baking sheet with foil and place the potatoes on the sheet.

2. Bake the potatoes in the oven for about an hour, or until the tender and cooked through. Remove from the oven and let it rest to cool before peeling and mashing. Once the potatoes have cooled, peel and mash in a mixing bowl. Set aside.

3. Reduce the oven to a temperature 350°F.

4. In the bowl with the mashed potatoes, mix in the cream, butter, maple syrup, almond extract, allspice, cinnamon and egg. Season to taste with salt and pepper and transfer into a greased baking dish, top with walnuts.

5. Bake it in the oven for about 20 to 25 minutes, or until the top is golden brown and cooked through. Remove from the oven and transfer into a wire rack, let it stand for 5 minutes before serving. Slice and serve.

Notes

OILY FISH

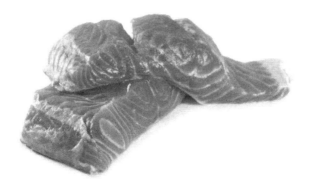

If you don't eat much fish, you might want to reconsider your diet. Fatty fish in particular is rich in DHA, a special fatty acid that's also found in your eye's retina. Research shows that low levels of DHA in the eye can lead to dry eyes and dry eye syndrome. So, if you possibly want to avoid refractive surgery in the future, eat more salmon, mackerel, tuna, trout, and anchovies. If you're one of these people who don't like fish, it's essential to take capsules containing omega-3 essential fatty acid to prevent dryness of the eyes.

SALMON WITH ROASTED RED PEPPERS

Ingredients:

- ¼ cup walnuts

- 1 garlic clove, minced

- ½ cup canned roasted bell peppers, drained

- 4 salmon fish fillets

- 1/2 teaspoon salt, divided

- Salt and coarsely ground black pepper, to taste

- 1 tablespoon tomato paste

- 1 teaspoon coconut oil

- Coconut oil, for greasing

Directions:

1. Apply medium-high heat to a lightly greased pan.

2. Season fillets with salt and pepper, place fillets on the pan and pan fry for about 4

to 5 minutes on each side. Carefully flip it over to cook the other side of the fillets. Cook for another 4 minutes or until the fish is flaky when tested with a fork. Remove from heat and set aside.

3. While cooking the fillets, combine together the tomato paste, garlic, walnuts, ¼ teaspoon salt, black pepper and roasted peppers in mixing bowl in blender or food processor. Pulse mixture until a smooth and thick consistency is achieved.

4. Place the fish on a serving dish, spoon over pesto sauce on top and then serve.

Notes

POACHED TROUT

Ingredients:

- 6 cups of fish stock or water

- 1 cup apple cider vinegar

- 1 tablespoon whole peppercorns

- 1 bay leaf

- 1 medium carrot, peeled and diced

- 1 stem of leek, roughly chopped

- 2 fresh Trout fish, filleted or butterflied

- Spring onions, chopped for garnish

- ¼ cup of coconut oil

Directions:

1. In a stockpot over high heat, add the stock, apple cider vinegar, chopped leek, whole peppercorns, bay leaf and diced carrot. Cover with lid and bring to a boil. Reduce to low heat and simmer for 10 minutes.

2. Poach in the trout for 10 minutes in the boiling stock. Remove fish with a slotted spoon and transfer into a serving dish. Set aside.

3. In mixing bowl, whisk together ¼ cup of the poaching liquid and the coconut oil. Pour mixture in top of the poached Trout fish. Serve with chopped spring onions and extra black pepper on top.

Notes

FENNEL PASTA WITH SARDINES AND PUMPKIN NUTS

Ingredients:

- 2 tablespoons coconut oil

- 1/4 cup chopped walnuts, toasted

- ½ kg gluten-free penne pasta or any short pasta

- 1 medium white onion, minced

- 2 fennel bulbs, trimmed and thinly sliced

- 1 tablespoon of garlic, minced

- 1 teaspoon salt, or as needed to taste

- ¼ teaspoon black pepper, freshly ground to taste

- 8 pieces of canned sardines in oil, drained

- 1 organic lemon, juiced and zested

- 1 organic lemon, sliced into rounds for serving

Directions:

1. Bring a large pot with water to a boil. Cook gluten-free pasta according to package directions or until al dente, approximately for 8 minutes. Drain and set aside.

2. While cooking the pasta, lightly toast the walnuts in a hot pan with oil for 4 minutes, or until fragrant. Stir in the garlic, onions, sliced fennel bulbs and season to taste with salt and pepper. Cook for about 8 to 10 minutes until the ingredients are soft and fragrant while stirring occasionally. Stir in the sardines, lemon zest, lemon juice and cook for another 5 minutes while stirring occasionally.

3. Stir in the cooked pasta and ¼ cup of the cooking liquid, cook for 2 to 3

minutes or until the sauce has reduced and thickened. Remove from heat.

4. Portion into individual serving plates, top with extra lemon zest and serve immediately.

Notes

WHOLE GRAIN

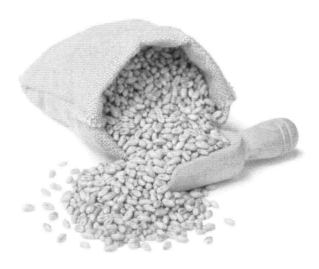

Wholes grains have always been promoted as the 'healthy' food, but we're never really told why. A diet that has a low glycemic index (GI) will dramatically reduce your risk of developing any eye condition related to ageing such as macular degeneration. Additionally, whole grains contain an impressive amount of vitamin E, niacin and zinc, which together will help with you overall eye health. Ditch the refined carbs in your diet such as white breads and pasta and opt for brown rice, oats, whole-wheat breads, and quinoa instead.

BLUEBERRY-BARLEY GRANOLA

Ingredients:

- 1/3 cup local honey

- 2 tablespoons raw cane sugar

- 2 tablespoons coconut oil

- ½ cup organic mixed seeds

- 2 cups rolled barley flakes

- ½ tablespoon of cinnamon

- ½ cup dried blueberries

- 1 1/2 teaspoons almond extract

- 1/4 teaspoon salt

- A pinch of cardamom

- 1/4 cup oat bran

Directions:

1. Preheat oven to 325°F.

2. Line a baking sheet with parchment and then place the mixed seeds. Bake it in the oven for 5 minutes, or until lightly

toasted and fragrant. Remove from the oven and transfer on a wire rack to cool.

3. In a mixing bowl, combine together the honey, almond extract, salt, cardamom, cinnamon, oil and sugar. Mix in the oat bran and barley; continue mixing until the ingredients are evenly distributed.

4. Transfer mixture on the baking sheet with parchment paper and bake it in the oven for 20 to 25 minutes, or until lightly browned. Stir the mixture after the first 10 minutes of baking.

5. Remove from the oven and transfer on a wire rack to cool. Stir in the blueberries, transfer into a covered container and slice to serve.

Notes

WHEAT SALAD WITH BERRIES AND BACON

Ingredients:

- ½ cup walnuts, chopped

- 1 cup wheat berries

- 4 strips bacon

- ½ cup dried cherries

- ½ cup fresh flat-leaf parsley

- salt and black pepper, to taste

- 2 shallots, thinly sliced

- 2 tablespoons coconut oil

- 1 organic lemon, juiced

Directions:

1. In a large pan over medium-high heat, add 2 litres of water and bring it to a boil. Add salt and boil the wheat berries for about an hour, or until chewy. Rinse with cool running water and drain. Transfer into a bowl and set aside.

2. While boiling the wheat, preheat an oven to a temperature of 350° F. Place the walnut on a baking sheet and toast it in the oven for 8 to 10 minutes, or until lightly toasted and fragrant. Remove from the oven and let it rest to cool. Chop the walnuts and set aside.

3. In a pan skillet over medium-high heat, add the bacon and cook for about 5 to 7 minutes or until crispy. Place it on a plate with paper towels to drain the excess oil and to cool. Chop the bacon, transfer into the bowl with the wheat berries and stir in the walnuts, shallots, cherries, oil, parsley and lemon juice. Season to taste with salt and ground pepper, and then gently toss the ingredients to combine.

4. Portion into individual serving bowls and serve immediately.

Notes

WHOLE GRAIN GRANOLA

Ingredients:

- 2 cups rolled barley

- 1 ½ cups organic mixed nuts

- 2 ½ cups Khorasan wheat

- 1 cup shredded coconut

- 1 cup organic mixed seeds

- ½ cup honey

- ½ tablespoon salt

- ½ cup coconut oil

- 1/3 cup raw cane sugar

Directions:

1. Preheat an oven to a temperature of 300°F. Line a baking sheet with parchment paper, set aside.

2. In a mixing bowl, add and mix all ingredients until evenly distributed. Place it on the baking sheet and bake for

about 30 minutes. Stir the mixture after the first 10 minutes in the oven, and then stir again after 20 minutes.

3. Remove from the oven, transfer into a wire rack to cool before serving.

Notes

LEGUMES

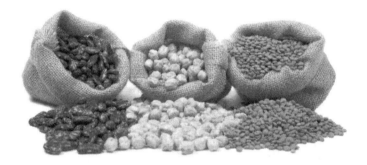

Legumes are powerful sources of nutrition, and they provide your body with an excellent dose of zinc and bioflavonoids, which help protect the eye's retina. It also reduces the risk of developing any age-related eye condition in the future such as macular degeneration and cataracts. Countries in the Middle East and the Mediterranean, where diets are high in lentils, haricot beans, kidney beans, and black-eyed peas, have lower rates of cataracts than countries that diets don't include such high amount of legumes.

BLACK BEANS CHEESY CHICKEN QUESADILLAS

Ingredients:

- 2 large red bell pepper, seeded and diced

- 4 stems of spring onions, thinly sliced

- 2 cups cooked organic chicken, shredded

- 1 cup canned black beans, rinsed and drained

- ½ cup cooked plain white rice or brown rice

- ½ cup sour cream

- 8 gluten-free corn tortillas for burritos

- 2 cups Parmesan cheese, shredded

- 1 teaspoon coconut oil

- Coconut oil, for greasing

- 1 cup of any homemade or readymade salsa

Directions:

1. In a mixing bowl, combine together the shredded chicken, cooked rice, spring onions, beans and bell pepper. Place the tortilla on a flat work surface, portion the chicken mixture and cheese on top of each tortilla. Fold each tortilla and press down to seal the edges. Lightly brush stuffed tortillas with oil, set aside.

2. In a wide skillet over medium-low heat, cook two stuffed tortillas with the oiled side down. Cook for about 5 minutes on each side or until golden brown, flip tortillas to cook the other side. Cook the remaining tortillas and transfer to a plate.

3. Cut the tortillas into wedges or into half and serve with sour cream and salsa on the side.

Notes

PASTA E FAGIOLI

Ingredients:

- 3 to 4 links of Italian sausage, cooked ahead then chopped

- 1 tablespoon coconut oil

- 1 medium white onion, minced

- 2 garlic cloves, minced

- 1 teaspoon thyme, dried

- ½ teaspoon rosemary, dried

- 4 cups low-sodium organic chicken broth

- ½ cup gluten-free elbow pasta (about 250 g)

- 1 cup canned chickpeas, rinsed and drained

- 1 cup canned crushed tomatoes

- ¼ cup Parmesan cheese, grated

- fresh thyme and crushed red pepper flakes, to taste

Directions:

1. In a stockpot over medium-high heat, add in the oil. Once the oil is hot, sauté the onions for 3 minutes, stir in the garlic. Cook for 3 minutes while stirring occasionally. Stir in dried thyme, rosemary and 3 ½ cups organic chicken broth.

2. Bring it to a boil and stir in the pasta. Cook the pasta for about 6 to 8 minutes or until firm to the bite.

3. While cooking the pasta, add the remaining broth, chickpeas and tomatoes. Pulse ingredients until smooth and thick. Pour puree into the stockpot together with the chopped sausage. Return to a boil, reduce heat to low and simmer for 10 minutes.

4. Portion soup into individual serving
bowls and top with grated Parmesan,
thyme and red pepper flakes.

Notes

BUTTER-BEAN ALMOND CUP CAKES

Ingredients:

- ¼ cup of almonds, chopped

- 2 organic eggs

- 1 teaspoon of baking powder

- 1 teaspoon of baking soda

- ¼ cup of raw cane sugar

- ½ cup of grass-fed butter, unsalted

- 1 cup of Fava beans, cooked

- ¼ cup of walnuts, chopped

- 3 packets of stevia

- 4 tablespoons of Tahini sauce

- Arrowroot-stevia mixture (½ packet stevia and ¼ cup arrowroot flour mixture)

- 2 teaspoons of coconut milk

Directions:

1. In a pan over medium- high heat, add and boil 2 cups of water and cook the fava beans for 5 to 7 minutes. Remove from heat and transfer into a plate, discarding the cooking liquid.

2. Combine the almonds, fava beans, cane sugar and eggs in food processor. Pulse into a coarse mixture and stir in the tahini sauce, baking powder and baking soda. Pulse again until a smooth and thick consistency is achieved.

3. Preheat an oven to a temperature of 350°F and place paper cups on a muffin tray, set aside.

4. Transfer mixture into mixing bowl and mix in the chopped walnuts. Pour the mixture in the paper cups and bake it in the oven for 15 minutes.

5. While baking the cupcakes, soften butter in a mixing bowl and mix in half of the arrowroot-stevia mixture. Whisk ingredients thoroughly until smooth and creamy. Whisk in the remaining arrowroot-stevia mixture and the coconut milk. Whisk thoroughly until well combined.

6. When the cupcakes are done, remove from the oven, transfer on a wire rack and let it stand for 5 minutes to cool.

7. Place the butter-milk mixture on a pipe bag and pipe mixture on top of each cupcake and then serve.

Notes

GRASS FED BEEF

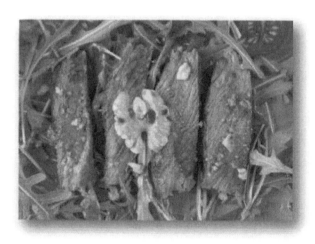

Dismiss any information that tells you beef is unhealthy. When eaten in moderation, beef can boost your health ten-fold, especially your eye health. Always opt for the leaner, grass fed versions, but beef in general has high amounts of zinc. Zinc works together with vitamin A, a vitamin essential for eye health. Zinc helps assist the absorption of vitamin A, so essentially vitamin A is useless without zinc. With the combination of vitamin A and zinc, you'll help reduce the risk of any age-related eye conditions, such as macular degeneration.

THAI COCONUT BEEF IN CRISPY WONTON CUPS

Ingredients:

For the beef

- ¼ cup coconut oil

- 1 pound grass-fed beef brisket, cut into cubes

- 1 cup of coconut milk

- 4 tablespoons red Thai curry paste

- ¼ cup Tamari soy sauce

- 2 tablespoons rice vinegar

- 2 tablespoons hot chili sauce

- 1 organic lime, sliced into rounds

- 1 stalk of lemon grass, finely chopped

- 1-inch of fresh ginger root, minced

- 4 garlic cloves, crushed

- Salt and coarsely ground pepper, to taste

- Fresh Cilantro leaves, for garnish

- Organic beef broth, as need

For the wonton cups

- Square gluten-free wonton wrappers

- oil

- toasted sesame seeds

- salt

Directions:

1. Cut the beef into large cubes, generously season with salt and pepper and set aside.

2. In a large pot over high heat, add in the oil. Once the oil is hot, sear the sides of the beef until browned. In order to achieve a nice sear of the beef, cook them by batch. When the beef edges starts to brown, turn to cook the sear the other sides. Remove from pot and continue to cook the remaining beef.

3. Deglaze the pot with coconut milk, scraping the bottom and sides to remove brown bits to add flavor to the dish. Add the remaining ingredients for the beef and bring to a boil while stirring occasionally.

4. Return the seared beef and place them in a single layer. Slowly add beef broth until beef is covered in 3/4.

5. Place beef back in the pan in a single layer. Add enough water so that the beef is ¾ covered with liquid. Cover lid and reduce to low heat when the cooking liquid starts to bubble, simmer for 4 to 5 hours or until the beef is tender.

6. When the beef is done, with a slotted spoon remove from the cooking liquid, transfer into a plate to cool. Increase the heat and cook the sauce until it has reduced in half.

7. Shred the beef and return to the pot with the sauce, season to taste with salt and pepper. Toss beef to coat and set aside.

For the wonton

1. Separate wonton wrappers and lay them in a floured work surface. Lightly brush the top part with oil, sprinkle with sesame seed on the edges and sprinkle with small amount of salt.

2. With your thumb and index finger, press the each corner to form like cups. Place the wrappers in a greased baking sheet and bake it in the oven for about 3 to 4 minutes.

3. Remove from the oven and cool on a wire rack. Serve Thai Coconut Beef with crispy wonton cups.

Notes

THAI BEEF SALAD

Ingredients:

- 1 cup loosely packed fresh mint leaves

- 1 cup loosely packed fresh basil leaves

- 1 large purple onion, halved and thinly sliced

- Salt and coarsely ground black pepper, to taste

- 8 organic kaffir leaves, cut into chiffonades

- 3 red hot chili pepper, seeded and minced

- 2 pounds grass-fed beef sirloin steaks, excess fat trimmed

- 2 cups of loosely packed mixed salad greens

- 1 cup loosely packed fresh coriander leaves

For dressing

- 2 tablespoons fish sauce

- 2 organic limes, juiced

- 1 teaspoon Tamari soy sauce

- 3 packets stevia

Directions:

1. Lightly brush the beef steaks with oil and season with salt and pepper.

2. Preheat a gas grill with high heat and brush the grates with oil. Reduce heat to medium-low and grill the steaks, turning once to cook the other side until medium-well. Remove from grill, transfer on a plate and let it stand for 5 minutes. Thinly slice the meat and set aside.

3. In a large mixing bowl, add the mixed greens, lime leaves, onions, chili, mint, cilantro and basil. Gently toss and set aside.

4. Combine the stevia, soy sauce, fish sauce and lime juice in a small bowl. Whisk it thoroughly until the stevia is completely dissolved.

5. Portion salad on individual serving bowls, top each bowl with sliced beef and drizzle with salad dressing on top. Serve immediately.

Notes

SMOKED BBQ BEEF SANDWICHES WITH COOL RANCH COLESLAW

Ingredients:

Bbq Beef

- 2 tablespoons grass-fed butter

- 1 large onion, chopped

- 2 cups of Bbq sauce

- 4 pounds boneless grass-fed beef chuck roast

- ¼ cup of any spice rub mixture

- ¼ cup white vinegar

- ½ cup apple juice

- ¼ cup Worcestershire Sauce

- ½ teaspoon garlic powder

- ½ teaspoon onion powder

- 1 teaspoon chili powder

- 1 teaspoon black pepper, coarsely ground

- ¼ cup raw cane sugar

- 1 tablespoon yellow mustard

Coleslaw

- 1/2 teaspoon onion powder

- ¼ teaspoon ground pepper, to taste

- 1 to 1/2 cup mayonnaise

- ¼ teaspoon garlic salt

- ¼ teaspoon onion salt

- 1 cup sour cream

- 1 bag coleslaw mix

- 3 tablespoons whites vinegar

- 1 tablespoon fresh chives, chopped

- 1 tablespoon fresh parsley leaves, chopped

- 1 ½ packet stevia

Directions:

1. Rub the meat with the spice rub. Smoke until medium rare or medium well. Place the meat in a slow cooker and cook on low for 4 hours, or until tender and it can be easily pulled apart. When beef is done shred with 2 forks and remove any fat. Set aside.

2. Melt grass-fed butter in a saucepan over a medium low heat, add onions. Cook until the onions are soft and translucent, or for about 5 minutes.

3. Add the remaining ingredients for the Bbq beef ingredients and simmer for 30 minutes.

4. Transfer the shredded beef in a large mixing bowl and pour over the BBQ sauce. Toss ingredients to coat beef evenly with the sauce. Set aside.

5. To make the coleslaw, combine all ingredients except for the coleslaw mix. Once the ingredients are well incorporated, add the coleslaw mix and mix well. Set aside.

6. Reheat the Bbq if chilled and place it in a serving bowl, serve with assorted bread rolls and coleslaw in a separate bowl.

Notes

COCONUT MILK

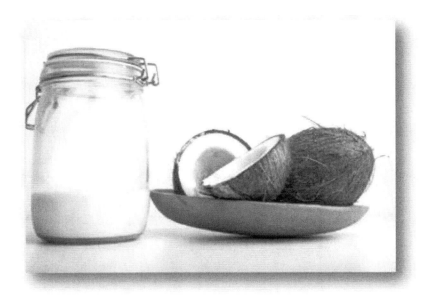

Coconut milk is full of amazingly helpful medium chain triglycerides that has a laundry list of beneficial effects including:

1. An additional energy source for brain function which includes the visual center.

2. Antimicrobial effects fighting of these viruses:

   HIV

measles

herpes simplex (HSV-1)

vesicular stomatitis virus

visna virus

cytomegalovirus (CMV)

3. All natural SunScreen

These are just a few of the amazing characteristics of coconut, coconut oil and coconut milk.

COCONUT MILK SMOOTHIE

Ingredients:

- 1 cup canned coconut milk

- 2 tablespoons of honey or 3 packets of stevia

- 1 cup frozen blueberries

- 2 ripe bananas, peeled and sliced

- 1 cup low-fat yogurt

Directions:

1. Chop the peeled bananas, blueberries and transfer in blender together with the coconut milk, yogurt and honey. Pulse mixture until smooth and creamy.

2. Portion smoothie on serving glasses, serve immediately.

Notes

THAI GREEN CHICKEN CURRY

Ingredients:

- 1 tablespoon coconut oil

- 1 ½ tablespoons green curry paste

- 6 organic chicken thighs, skinned and deboned, cut into strips

- 2 cups of coconut milk

- 3 lime leaves, chopped

- 2 tablespoons light soy sauce

- 1 tablespoon raw cane sugar

- ½ pound green beans, trimmed and cut into bias

- ½ pound asparagus spears, trimmed and cut into bias

- salt and freshly ground black pepper, to taste

For serving

- Thai fragrant rice or any gluten-free rice, cooked ahead according to package directions

- 1 cup loosely packed fresh coriander leaves, roughly chopped

Directions:

1. In a wok over high heat, add in the oil. Once the oil is very hoe and smoking, add the green curry paste and cook for 2 minutes while stirring occasionally.

2. Stir in the chicken and toss to coat evenly with curry paste. Stir-fry for 2 to 3 minutes until the chicken is lightly browned.

3. Add the chopped lime leaves, light soy sauce and sugar and then stir it well. Cover with lid and bring it to a boil. Reduce to low heat and simmer for 10 minutes, or until the liquid has thickened.

4. Add the asparagus and green beans and simmer for 4 minutes while stirring occasionally. Season to taste with salt and pepper and remove from heat.

5. Portion rice into individual serving bowls, top with chicken and ladle over with green curry sauce. Serve with coriander leaves on top.

Notes

SLOW-COOKED BUTTER CHICKEN

Ingredients:

- 3 tablespoons grass-fed butter

- 2 tablespoons coconut oil

- 3 cloves garlic, minced

- 2 tablespoons red curry paste

- 4 organic chicken thighs, skinned and deboned, cubed

- 1 medium white onion, diced

- 1 tablespoon curry powder

- 1 tablespoon garam masala

- 1 cup canned stewed tomatoes

- 8 pods of green cardamom

- 2 cups of coconut milk

- 1 cup low fat yoghurt

- Salt, to taste

Directions:

1. In a large pan over medium heat, melt in the butter and stir in the onion, garlic and cubed chicken. Cook for about 10 minutes or until the vegetables are soft and fragrant. Stir in the red curry paste, curry powder, garam masala and stewed tomatoes and cook for about 5 minutes.

2. Remove from heat and transfer into slow cooker. Stir in the yogurt, coconut milk and cardamom pods. Season to taste with salt and pepper.

3. Cook chicken on low for about 6 to 8 hours, or 4 to 6 hours on high. Once the chicken is tender and the sauce has thickened, remove from slow cooker and transfer into a serving bowl or dish, remove and discard cardamom pods.

Notes

TOMATOES

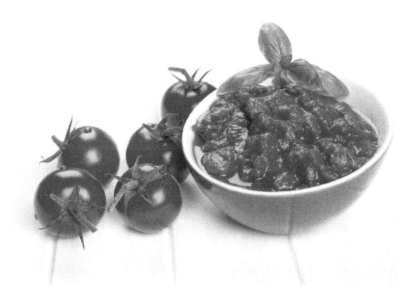

Tomatoes may just be that simple red fruit you find in your salad, but these fruits are packed with carotenoids, which are responsible for the tomato's bright red color. Lycopene, which is one of the important cartenoids in tomatoes, helps promote the eyes' ocular tissues and helps reduce any light-induced damage to the eye's retina.

TOMATO AND PEACH SALAD

Ingredients:

- 2 ripe peaches, pitted and cut into wedges,

- 1 cup ripe red tomatoes, cut into wedges

- 1 cup cherry tomatoes, halved

- 2 red onions, halved and then thinly sliced

- 1 tablespoon white wine vinegar

- 1 tablespoon coconut oil

- 1/4 cup goat's cheese or any soft cheese, crumbled

- ¼ cup loosely packed fresh basil leaves

- 1 packet of stevia

- Salt and freshly ground black pepper, to taste

Directions:

1. In a large mixing bowl, combine together the peach wedges, tomato

wedges, halved cherry tomatoes and sliced onions. Set aside.

2. In a separate mixing bowl, whisk together the wine vinegar, stevia, coconut oil, and a pinch of salt and pepper. Whisk the ingredients thoroughly and drizzle it on top of the fresh salad ingredients. Top with crumbled cheese and basil on top, serve immediately.

Notes

CREAMY PESTO CHICKEN

Ingredients

- 4 organic chicken breast fillets

- 3 tablespoons of homemade pesto

- ½ cup cream cheese

- 4 tablespoons coconut oil

- ½ cup coconut crumbs

- 1 cup tomatoes, halved

- 1 organic egg, beaten

- handful almonds, toasted and chopped

- handful basil leaves

Directions:

1. Preheat and oven to a temperature of 400°F. Lightly grease a baking sheet and set aside.

2. Make a shallow incision along the side of the breast fillets to form a pocket.

3. In a mixing bowl, mix together the pesto sauce and cream cheese until combined. Stuff breast fillets with pesto cheese mixture and level the opening with a spatula to seal. Lightly brush the breast fillets with oil and season with salt and pepper.

4. Mix the coconut crumbs with salt and pepper on a plate. Place the beaten egg on a separate small bowl. Coat the breast with egg and dredge evenly with seasoned coconut crumbs. Transfer the coated breasts on the greased baking sheet and place the tomatoes on the sides. Drizzle with the remaining oil on top.

5. Bake it in the preheated oven for about 20 to 25 minutes or until golden brown and cooked through. Before removing the breast from the oven, place the

almonds on the baking sheet and bake for another 2 to 3 minutes.

6.   Remove from the oven and transfer into a serving dish. Place the tomatoes on the side and top with toasted almonds and basil. Serve immediately.

Notes

RED AND YELLOW TOMATO GAZPACHO

Ingredients:

- 2 cups of ripe yellow tomatoes concasse, core removed

- 2 cups ripe red tomatoes concasse, core removed

- 1 large cucumber, peeled and seeded

- 1 cup cherry tomatoes, halved

- 1 garlic clove, minced

- 2 teaspoons red wine vinegar

- 1 ½ teaspoons balsamic vinegar

- 1 ½ teaspoons salt

- 5 tablespoons coconut oil

- Black pepper, freshly ground

- 2 boiled organic eggs, chopped, for garnish

- 4 strips crispy bacon, chopped for garnish

Directions:

1. In a pot with 2 litres of water, apply high heat and bring to a boil.

2. Remove the core of each red and yellow tomato and make a cross cut on the opposite side of the core. Blanche the tomatoes in the pot with boiling water for about 2 to 3 minutes, or until the skin starts to separate from the flesh. Remove with a slotted spoon and transfer in large bowl with ice bath. Peel the tomatoes and remove the seeds, finely chop and transfer in a large mixing bowl. Set aside.

3. Finely grate the cucumber and place it in the bowl with the tomatoes. Stir in the cherry tomatoes, vinegar, garlic and season to taste with salt and pepper.

4. Puree the ingredients in a blender until smooth and return to the bowl. Cover

and chill for at least 1 hour before serving.

5. Portion into individual serving bowls. Serve with bacon bits and chopped eggs on top.

Notes

OLIVE OIL

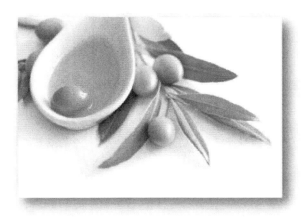

Olive oil is not just a dressing for your salad or a healthy way of frying it's also a great way to help protect your eyes' health. When you consciously follow a diet that has a low amount of trans and saturated fats, you'll reduce the risk of contracting retina diseases. Research also shows it helps reduce the risk of ARMD by a whopping 48%. If you're buying olive oil, make sure you go for the extra virgin version as this contains more antioxidants.

OLIVE OIL AND LEMON PASTA

Ingredients:

- 1 pound gluten-free spaghetti/linguine

- ¼ cup Parmesan cheese, grated

- 2 organic lemons, juiced and zested

- ¼ cup olive oil

- 2 garlic cloves, minced

- ½ cup stuffed olives, sliced

- 1 cup cherry tomatoes, halved

- ¼ cup basil, chopped

- salt and freshly ground black pepper, to taste

Directions:

1. In a mixing bowl, combine together the garlic, stuffed olives, cherry tomatoes, lemon zest, lemon juice, and olive oil. Set aside.

2. In a pot with boiling water, cook the gluten free pasta until firm to the bite. Drain and place it in a bowl, reserve ¼ cup of the cooking liquid.

3. Toss in the pasta with in the bowl with dressing and add ¼ cup of cooking liquid.

4. Add the chopped basil and grated Parmesan, season to taste with salt and pepper and gently toss to coat pasta evenly with dressing.

5. Portion pasta into individual serving bowls and serve with extra grated Parmesan on top.

Notes

ROASTED ASPARAGUS WITH LEMON

Ingredients:

- 1 tablespoon organic lemon juice

- 3 tablespoons of extra virgin olive oil

- ¼ cup of Parmesan cheese, grated

- 1 garlic clove, minced

- ½ pound of asparagus spears, trimmed

- 1 teaspoon salt, to taste

- 1/2 teaspoon black pepper, coarsely ground

Directions:

1. Preheat an oven to a temperature of 425 °F. Lightly grease a baking sheet and set aside.

2. In a mixing bowl, add the trimmed asparagus and add the oil. Add in the minced garlic, grated Parmesan, and gently toss to coat the asparagus. Season

with salt and black pepper, toss again and transfer on the greased baking sheet.

3. Bake it in the oven for about 15 minutes or until the asparagus are tender and cooked. Remove from the oven and transfer into a serving bowl or plate.

4. Drizzle with lemon juice, briefly toss and serve immediately.

Notes

ROSEMARY AND GRAPEFRUIT OLIVE OIL CAKE

Ingredients:

- 4 organic eggs, quartered

- 6 tablespoons olive oil

- 1 small grapefruit, peeled and segmented

- 2 ½ cups raw cane sugar

- 3 cups coconut flour, sifted

- 2 teaspoons baking powder

- 1 teaspoon baking soda

- 1 teaspoon salt

- Sprig fresh rosemary, chopped

- Arrowroot-stevia mixture (½ packet stevia and ¼ cup arrowroot flour mixture)

Directions:

1. In a pot over medium heat, add 3 cups of water, segmented grapefruit, 1 cup of

sugar and cook for 25 to 30 minutes while stirring occasionally. Remove grapefruit from the pot, place it in a bowl and reserve the cooking liquid.

2. Preheat and oven to a temperature of 350° F. Lightly grease a round baking pan and set aside.

3. In a mixing bowl, combine together the coconut flour, salt, baking powder, baking soda and the chopped rosemary. Set aside.

4. In a food processor, add in the grapefruit, the eggs the remaining sugar, oil and half the flour. Pulse until the ingredients are evenly distributed, add the remaining flour and briefly pulse again just to combine the ingredients. Do not over mix.

5. Place the mixture into the greased baking pan and bake it in the oven for about 40 to 45 minutes. It is done when a toothpick inserted in the thickest part comes out clean. Remove from the oven and transfer on a wire to cool. Lightly brush the top with the reserved cooking liquid, let it stand for 10 minutes before serving.

6. Remove from pan and transfer on a serving plate, dust heavily with arrowroot-stevia mixture. Serve.

Notes

NON-GMO CORN

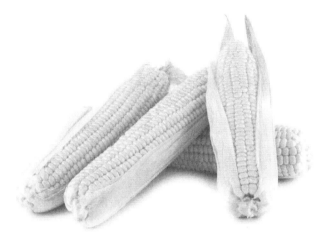

If you're a corn lover, you're in luck. Corn has high amounts of lutein and zeaxanthin, and only ½ a cup of boiled corn contains 1.8g of healthy pigments per serving. The pigments that are found in corn are also naturally occurring in the eye, but when ARMD sets in, these pigments are lost. When you eat more foods that contain such rich pigments, you significantly reduce the risk of losing your eyes' natural pigments.

NON-GMO CORN AVOCADO SALAD

Ingredients:

- 1 avocado, pitted and diced

- 2 ripe red tomatoes, diced

- 2 yellow tomatoes, diced

- 4 ears of non-GMO corn, cooked and removed from the cob

- ½ cup loosely packed fresh basil leaves, chopped

- 3 to 4 garlic cloves, minced

- 2 organic limes, juiced

- Salt and ground pepper, to taste

Directions:

1. In a mixing bowl, combine together all ingredients and then season to taste with salt and pepper. Gently toss to combine.

2. Portion salad into individual serving bowls or plates, drizzle with extra lemon juice if preferred and serve immediately.

Notes

NON-GMO CORN AND BLACK BEAN SALSA

Ingredients:

- 2 cups canned black beans, drained
- 1 cup cherry tomatoes, halved
- 1 red hot chili pepper, chopped
- 2 medium purple onion, diced
- 2 tablespoons of hot chili sauce
- 2 cups frozen non-GMO corn, thawed
- 3 teaspoon garlic, minced
- 1 cup loosely packed cilantro, chopped
- 2 tablespoons sherry vinegar
- 1 teaspoon chili powder, as needed for extra heat (optional)
- ½ teaspoon cumin
- 3 organic lime, juiced
- 2 teaspoons salt
- 1 teaspoon black pepper, freshly ground

Directions:

1. In a mixing bowl, add and mix the beans and corn. Set aside.

2. Dice the onions and chop the garlic, chili and cilantro and place it in a separate bowl. Add the remaining ingredients, toss to combine.

3. In the bowl with the corn-bean mixture, add in the mixed ingredients and toss again to coat the corn and beans with the dressing. Chill for an hour before serving.

Notes

CHILI BEEF WITH NON-GMO CORN

Ingredients:

- 1 tablespoon coconut oil

- 2 carrots, peeled and cubed

- 1 onion, diced

- 1 red bell pepper, diced

- ½ pound grass-fed beef, ground

- 2 tablespoons tomato paste

- 2 cups canned black beans, drained

- 1 red hot chili pepper

- salt and coarsely ground black pepper, to taste

- 1 cup of non-GMO corn kernels, thawed if frozen

- ½ cup Parmesan cheese, grated

- 2 scallions, chopped

- 3 cups of organic beef stock

Directions:

1. In a large pan over medium-high heat, add in the oil. Once the oil is hot, sauté in the onion, carrots, bell pepper and chili pepper for 3 minutes while stirring occasionally.

2. Stir in the ground beef and cook for 5 minutes while breaking up the meat with a wooden spoon.

3. Stir in the tomato paste and cook for 2 minutes or until the color has darkened a bit.

4. Add the beans, chili powder, beef stock and season to taste with salt and pepper. Cover lid and bring it to a boil. Reduce to low heat and simmer for 10 minutes. Add the corn just before removing the pan from heat.

5. Portion into individual serving bowls, serve with grated Parmesan and scallions on top.

Notes

PISTACHIOS

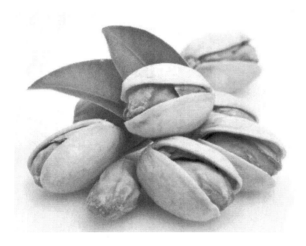

Although pistachios fall into the category of nuts, they're worthy of their own mention as they contain high amounts of zeaxanthin and lutein, which help restore the retina and ward off ARMD. Not only are they high in these antioxidants, they also contain high amounts of vitamin E and eating pistachios can reduce the risk of developing cataracts and other age-related eye diseases. If this isn't enough pistachios also contain mono and polyunsaturated fats that help accelerate the absorption of carotenoids, thus making the pistachio one of the healthiest snacks for your eyes.

SALMON WITH PISTACHIO CRUST WITH CREAMY LEMON SAUCE

Ingredients:

- 1 teaspoon salt

- ½ teaspoon black pepper, coarsely ground

- 1/4 cup cream

- 4 fresh salmon fillets

- 1/2 cup pistachio, chopped

For the sauce

- 1 cup heavy whipping cream

- 1 organic lemon, zested

- 1 shallot, minced

- 1 tablespoon coconut oil

- 1/4 teaspoon salt

- ¼ teaspoon cayenne pepper or a pinch of chili powder

Directions:

1. Preheat an oven to a temperature of 375°F. Lightly grease a baking sheet with oil, set aside.

2. Season salmon fillets with salt and pepper and place it on a greased baking sheet. Cover with cream and top with chopped pistachio on top.

3. Bake it in the oven for 15 to 20 minutes, or until it flakes easily when a fork is inserted and twisted on the flesh. Remove from the oven and set aside.

4. While cooking the fillets, apply medium-high heat on a small pan and add the oil. Once the oil is hot, sauté the shallots until soft and add the cream, lemon zest and cayenne pepper. Bring the mixture to a boil and then reduce to low heat. Simmer for 5 minutes or until the sauce

has thickened while stirring occasionally.

5. Place the sauce on a serving bowl and serve with the baked fish.

Notes

PISTACHIO BISCOTTI WITH CRANBERRIES

Ingredients:

- ½ tablespoon almond extract

- ½ cup dried cranberries

- ¼ cup coconut oil

- ¾ cup raw cane sugar

- 1 ½ cups pistachio nuts

- 2 organic eggs

- 1 ¾ cups coconut flour, sifted

- ¼ teaspoon salt

- 1 teaspoon baking powder

Directions:

1. Preheat an oven to a temperature of 300 °F. Line a baking sheet with parchment paper and set aside.

2. In a mixing bowl, mix together the oil and sugar until well incorporated. Stir in

the almond extract and eggs, and then whisk to combine.

3. In a separate bowl, combine the flour, salt and baking powder until evenly mixed. Gradually add it in the egg-sugar mixture, add the nuts and cranberries and mix it thoroughly.

4. Lightly kneads the dough mixture on a floured work surface and divide into 2 equal portions. Roll out the dough into 2-inch thick logs and transfer on a lined baking sheet.

5. Bake it in the oven for about 30 to 35 minutes, or until lightly browned. Remove from the oven and transfer on a wire rack, let it stand for 10 minutes.

6. Reduce oven temperature to 275 °F.

7. Slice the log on the diagonal into ¾ inch thick when it has lowered in

temperature. Return the slices on the baking sheet and bake for about 10 minutes or until brown and edges are crispy. Remove from the oven, transfer on a wire rack and let it stand for 5 minutes before serving.

Notes

PISTACHIO DARK GREEN LETTUCE SALAD

Ingredients:

- 1 cup canned mandarin oranges, drained

- 3 large heads of Dark green lettuce, torn or leaves separated

- 1 cup of pistachio, coarsely chopped

- 1 cup organic mixed dried fruits

For the dressing

- 2 tablespoons olive oil

- 1 packet of stevia

- ¼ cup rice vinegar

- ½ teaspoon salt

- ¼ teaspoon pepper, freshly ground

- 1-inch fresh ginger root, minced

Directions:

1. In a mixing bowl, mix together the pistachios, dried fruits, mandarin oranges and the lettuce. Set aside.

2. In food processor, add all of the dressing ingredients and pulse until smooth and well incorporated.

3. Drizzle the dressing on top of the fruit and lettuce mixture, gently toss to coat.

4. Serve with extra pistachios on top and cheese if preferred.

Notes

STRAWBERRIES

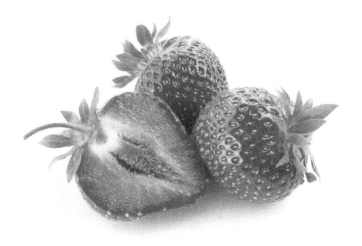

Who doesn't love this tasty summer fruit? Not only are strawberries the perfect partner for cream and ice-cream they also contain a number of beneficial nutrients to help you reach optimal eye health and sight. Strawberries have high amounts of vitamin C, which will help you fight and reduce inflammation of the eyes. It doesn't matter whether the inflammation is naturally occurring or self-inflicted from wearing makeup or your contacts too long, strawberries help reduce it. These red succulent berries also contain a variety of powerful antioxidants that will help your body defend your eyes when it comes to eye infections, dryness, and macular degeneration. All it takes is a cup of strawberries a day to help eliminate or prevent eye problems.

MOZZARELLA NAPOLEONS WITH STRAWBERRIES

Ingredients:

- 2 cups chopped fresh strawberries

- 3 sheets gluten-free phyllo dough, thawed if frozen

- 2 tablespoons grass-fed butter, melted

- 1 ½ teaspoons olive oil

- 2 tablespoons walnuts, toasted

- 2 tablespoons raw cane sugar

- 1 tablespoon of organic orange juice

- 3 packets of stevia

- 1 cup Mozzarella cheese, shredded

- 1 to 2 tablespoons of local honey

Directions:

1. Preheat oven to a temperature of 350°F. Line a baking sheet with parchment paper and set aside.

2. Finely chop the walnuts and place it in a bowl, mix in the sugar. Set aside. In a separate bowl, combine the butter and oil and set aside.

3. Place 1 dough on the baking sheet that is lined with parchment paper. Lightly brush with butter-oil mixture and top with half of the walnut-sugar mixture. Place dough on top and lightly brush again with butter-oil mixture, top with the remaining walnut-sugar mixture. Place the last dough on top, lightly brush with butter-oil mixture and dust with arrowroot-stevia mixture.

4. Divide the dough layers into quarters, and then dived each quarters into 3 portions. Separate the sliced doughs on the baking sheet, cover with parchment paper and place a baking sheet on top.

5. Bake it in the oven for about 10 to 12 minutes, or until golden brown. Remove the baking sheet on top, transfer on a wire and let it stand to cool.

6. In small bowl, combine together the cheese and honey. In a separate small bowl, coat strawberries with arrowroot-stevia mixture.

7. Place one slice of dough on each 4 serving plates, top with 1 tablespoon of cheese mixture and 2 tablespoons of coated strawberries. Repeat the procedure and finally cover with the remaining dough.

8. Serve immediately or chill.

Notes

CHICKEN SALAD WITH STRAWBERRIES

Ingredients:

Dressing

- 2 tablespoons olive oil

- 1 tablespoon raw cane sugar

- 2 tablespoons balsamic vinegar

- 1 tablespoon water

- Pinch of salt

- Pinch black pepper, freshly ground

Salad

- 1 large head of Romaine lettuce, torn or leaves separated

- 4 cups arugula

- 2 cups fresh or frozen strawberries, quartered

- 2 purple onion, chopped

- 1 organic chicken breast fillet, cooked ahead, diced or cut into strips

- 2 tablespoons walnuts, halved

- ½ cup of Gorgonzola cheese

Directions:

1. In a mixing bowl, whisk together all the dressing ingredients except for the oil. Gradually add in the oil and whisk until a smooth and thick consistency is achieved.

2. In a separate mixing bowl, combine the lettuce, arugula, strawberries, onions and chicken strips.

3. Portion salad into individual serving bowls and top with Gorgonzola cheese and walnuts. Drizzle the dressing over the salad and serve immediately.

Notes

SMOOTHIE BANANA-STRAWBERRIES

Ingredients:

- 1 ½ cups coconut milk

- 1 cup low fat yogurt

- 1 cup frozen fresh strawberries

- 1 banana, peeled and sliced

- 1 packet of stevia

Directions:

1. In a blender, add in the banana, strawberry, yogurt, coconut milk and stevia. Pulse blender until the mixture is smooth and creamy.

2. Portion into individual serving glasses. Serve immediately or chill for future consumption.

Notes

AVOCADO

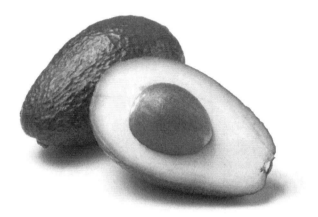

Toss it in a salad, spread it on toast or eat whole, when eaten raw, avocado provides your body with vitamins B6, C and E, all of which are essential for healthy eyesight. Avocado also helps reduce your stress levels, and while it's not directly related to your eyesight, stress has been proved to be one of the causes of vision loss.

SPICY SHRIMP-AVOCADO TORTILLA SOUP

Ingredients:

- 1 tablespoon coconut oil

- 2 large onions, diced

- 1 celery stalk, chopped

- 1 large carrot, peeled and diced

- 1 tablespoon red hot chili sauce

- ½ teaspoon cumin powder

- 1 teaspoon chili powder, or as preferred for extra heat

- 2 to 3 garlic cloves, minced

- 4 cups low-sodium organic chicken stock

- 1 cup canned stewed tomatoes

- ½ pound fresh medium shrimp, peeled and deveined

- 1 organic lime, juiced

- Pinch of salt, to taste

- ½ cup baked corn tortilla chips, lightly crushed

- 1 avocado, pitted and diced

- ½ cup loosely packed fresh cilantro leaves (optional)

Directions:

1. In a pan over medium-high heat, add in the oil and sauté the onions, garlic, celery, carrots, chili sauce, chili powder and cumin. Cook for about 5 minutes while stirring occasionally. Pour in the broth and tomatoes, cover lid and bring to a boil.

2. Stir in the shrimp and simmer for about 3 to 4 minutes, or until the shrimp is opaque and cooked through.

3. Stir in the lime juice and salt. Remove pan from heat.

4. Portion shrimp into individual serving bowls and top with tortillas and avocado. Serve with chopped cilantro if preferred.

Notes

AVOCADO AND PRAWN SALAD WITH CHILI-LIME DRESSING

Ingredients:

- ½ cup mixed salad greens

- 1 pound of cooked prawns, heads removed

- 2 avocados, pitted and sliced

- ½ cup tightly packed fresh basil leaves

For the dressing

- 1 red hot chilli, finely chopped

- 3 tablespoons olive oil

- 1 organic lime, sliced into wedges

- 1 organic lime, juiced

- 2 teaspoons clear honey

Directions:

1. Remove the heads of the prawns, rinse in cool running water and drain or pat dry with paper towels. Place it in a bowl and toss in the chopped basil. Set aside.

2. In a mixing bowl, combine together all ingredients and whisk until well incorporated.

3. In a separate bowl, add the sliced avocado and toss with half of the dressing.

4. Portion salad leaves on serving plates then top with the prawns. Serve with lime wedges and drizzle with dressing on top.

Notes

AVOCADO LIME CHEESECAKE TART

Ingredients:

- 1/3 cup raw cane sugar

- ¼ cup of grass-fed butter

- 1 cup of cream cheese

- 1 cup pureed avocado

- 1 tablespoon almond extract

- 2 packets of stevia

- 2 large organic eggs, lightly beaten

- ¼ cup of yogurt

- 1 organic lime, juiced and zested

- 1 ¾ cup coconut flour

- ¼ teaspoon salt, or as needed to taste

Directions:

1. Preheat an oven to a temperature of 350°F.

2. In a mixing bowl, combine together the flour, sugar, and ¼ teaspoon of salt. Fold in the butter until lumps form. Transfer into a tart pan and press down into the bottom. Bake it in the oven for about 10 to 15 minutes, or until lightly browned.

3. In a separate bowl, mix together the cheese, avocado puree, stevia until thick and fluffy. Add in the eggs, lime juice, lime zest, almond extract, yogurt and a pinch of salt. Whisk to combine.

4. Pour mixture in the pan with the crust and bake for about an hour. Remove from the oven, transfer on a wire rack and let it stand for 10 minutes. Chill for at least 2 hours before serving.

Notes

PEPPERS

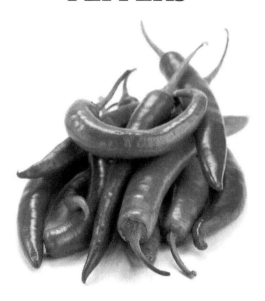

No matter what form or color your peppers come in, they're all beneficial to your eyes. Make eating all kinds of peppers of all colors a routine as they're one of the best sources of vitamins A and C. Peppers cooked or raw contain beta-carotene, vitamin B6, lutein, lycopene, and zeaxanthin, all of which help improve your eyesight.

ROASTED RED PEPPERS SALAD

Ingredients:

- 2 garlic cloves

- 1 tablespoon capers, rinsed

- 10 large bell peppers

- 1 to 2 teaspoons sherry vinegar

- Coconut oil, for greasing

- ½ cup stuffed olives, drained

- Fresh basil leaves, for garnish

- salt and freshly ground black pepper, to taste

Directions:

1. Char grill the bell peppers directly on top of the gas burner, use a thong to turn the peppers and to evenly roast the skin. When the skins are charred evenly, remove from the burner and transfer into a covered container to cool.

2. Cut the roasted bell peppers into half and remove the charred skin and seeds. Slice into long strips and place it in a bowl, season to taste with salt and pepper.

3. Crush the garlic with the flat side of a knife, sprinkle with salt and continue on crushing garlic into a paste. Stir in the garlic paste with the roasted peppers, together with the capers and sherry vinegar. Add in the oil and toss gently to combine.

4. Serve with extra salt and pepper if desired and top with olives and chopped basil.

Notes

MIXED BELL PEPPER STEAK

Ingredients:

- 2 teaspoons coconut oil

- 1 medium purple onion, thinly sliced

- 2 cloves garlic, minced

- 1 pound grass-fed beef top round steak, cut into thin strips

- 1 cup organic beef broth

- ¼ cup Tamari soy sauce

- ¼ teaspoon raw cane sugar

- ½ teaspoon black pepper, freshly ground

- 1 celery stalk, chopped

- 2 teaspoons arrowroot flour

- ¼ cup water

- 3 green bell pepper, sliced into long strips

- 3 red bell pepper, sliced into long strips

- 3 yellow bell pepper, sliced into long strips

- 1 cup of canned stewed tomatoes

Directions:

1. Slice the beef into long thin strips, set aside.

2. In a skillet over medium-heat, add in the oil. Once the oil is hot, sauté the onion and garlic until soft and fragrant, approximately 4 to 5 minutes. With a slotted spoon, remove sautéed ingredients from the skillet and place into a bowl. Set aside.

3. Add the beef in the skillet and sauté for about 5 to 7 minutes or until lightly brown, stirring occasionally. Remove from skillet with a slotted spoon, place in a bow and set aside.

4. Pour in the broth, tamari soy sauce, black pepper, cane sugar in the same skillet and ring to a boil.

5. Stir and return the onions, garlic and beef in the skillet and bring to a boil. Reduce to low heat and simmer for about 25 to 30 minutes. Add the chopped celery, stewed tomatoes and the bell peppers. Cover lid and simmer for another 5 minutes, or until the vegetables are cooked but crisp.

6. In a small bowl, completely dissolve the arrowroot flour with water and pour it in the skillet. Cook for another 2 minutes while stirring regularly.

7. Remove from heat and transfer into a serving bowl. Serve with extra chopped herbs on top if preferred.

Notes

SWEET SPICED ROASTED RED PEPPER WITH FETA HUMMUS

Ingredients:

- ½ cup canned roasted red peppers

- 2 organic lemon, juiced

- 1 ½ cup canned chickpeas, drained

- 1 ½ tablespoons sesame paste

- 1 garlic clove, minced

- ½ teaspoon cumin powder

- ½ cup goat's cheese, crumbled

- ½ teaspoon Spanish paprika

- ¼ teaspoon salt

- 1 tablespoon of minced fresh parsley

Directions:

1. In a food processor, add the chickpeas, roasted peppers, goat's cheese, lemon juice, sesame paste, garlic, smoked

paprika, cumin and salt. Pulse until a smooth consistency is achieved.

2. Place the pureed ingredients in a bowl and chill for at least 2 hours before serving.

3. Serve with chopped parsley on top.

Notes

DARK CHOCOLATE

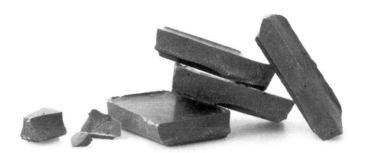

Rich in antioxidants, dark chocolate does wonders for your eyes. It is made up of powerful antioxidants like flavonols, which are known to enhance the blood flow to the eye's retina, thus helping your eyes to see evenly when the light is low.

DARK COCO-CHOCOLATE CAKE

Ingredients:

- ½ tablespoon baking powder

- ½ tablespoon baking soda

- ½ tablespoon of salt

- ¾ cup of baking cocoa

- 2 cups raw cane sugar

- 1 ¾ cup coconut flour, sifted

- 2 organic medium eggs

- 1 cup coconut milk

- ½ cup coconut oil

- 2 teaspoons almond extract

- 1 cup of boiling water, or as needed

Directions:

1. Preheat an oven to a temperature of 350°F. Lightly grease a 9 inch baking pan and lightly dust with flour. Set aside.

2. In a large bowl, whisk together the coconut milk, the almond extract, and the eggs until smooth.

3. In a separate bowl, combine all dry ingredients until evenly distributed.

4. Mix the dry and wet ingredients, and the gradually add in with ¾ cup of boiling water. Mix to combine and transfer into a greased and floured baking pan.

5. Bake it in the oven for about 30 to 35 minutes. It is done when a toothpick inserted in the thickest part comes out clean. Remove from the oven, transfer on a wire and let it stand for 10 minutes before serving and slicing.

Notes

EASY DARK WALNUT-CHOCOLATE CLUSTERS

Ingredients:

- 1 1/2 cups walnuts

- 1 cup melted dark chocolate

Directions:

1. Place a non-stick baking mat on a baking sheet.

2. Melt the dark chocolate on a double-boiler.

3. Take a tablespoon of melted chocolate and top with chopped or whole almonds. Repeat the procedure with the remaining ingredients.

4. Chill for at least 2 hours before serving.

Notes

KALE STRAWBERRY SALAD WITH CHOCO-VINAIGRETTE DRESSING

Ingredients:

Salad

- 1 medium cucumber, halved lengthwise and thinly sliced

- 1 cup of loosely packed kale

- 2 cups strawberries, halved

- ¼ cup Gorgonzola cheese, with black pepper, crumbled

Dressing

- ½ cup balsamic vinegar

- 6 packets of stevia

- ¼ cup of dark chocolate, cubed

Directions:

1. Portion kale leaves into individual serving plates, add cucumber slices,

Gorgonzola cheese, and strawberries on top.

2. In a mixing bowl, add and heat the balsamic vinegar and stevia until well combined. Remove from heat and melt in the dark chocolate. Drizzle the dressing on top of the salad ingredients and serve.

Notes

TEA AND COFFEE

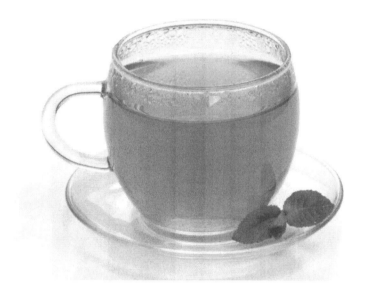

Tea and coffee may be surprising addition to the list to promote eye health, but research shows that drinking tea and coffee can assist in preventing macular degeneration, cataracts and dry eyes. Coffee and tea also stops the growth of new blood vessels towards the back of the eyes, which can cause vision loss if there's a buildup over time.

SPIKED SWEET LEMON TEA

Ingredients:

- 6 organic lemon, juiced

- 6 orange Pekoe tea bags

- 4 tablespoons of stevia

- 7 cups of water

- 1 cup rum

- Fresh mint leaves, for garnish

Directions:

1. Add 4 cups of water in a pot and apply high heat, bring to a boil and add the pekoe tea bags. Remove pot from heat, set aside and let it cool for about 10 minutes.

2. Remove the pekoe tea bags and discard, add the stevia and stir until completely dissolved. Stir in the organic lemon juice and rum.

3. Transfer into a covered container or pitcher and chill for at least 2 hours before serving.

4. Serve over ice, in tall glasses garnished with mint sprigs.

Notes

SLOW-COOKED COFFEE BRAISED SHORT RIBS

Ingredients:

- Salt and coarsely ground black pepper

- 2 tablespoons coconut oil

- 3 pounds grass-fed beef short ribs

- 1 cup Chardonnay

- 1 teaspoon oregano, dried

- 1 cup brewed coffee

- 1 large white onion, chopped

- 3 garlic cloves, crushed

- 1 tablespoon chili powder

Directions:

1. Rub the ribs evenly with salt and pepper. Set aside.

2. In a skillet over medium-high heat, add in the oil. Once the oil is hot, add the ribs and brown the sides for about 10

minutes, turning once too cook the other side. Transfer into plate lined with paper towels to drain excess fat.

3. Deglaze pan with wine and coffee, apply high heat and cook while scraping the brown bit on the bottom and sides. Cook until the sauce has reduced in half.

4. Transfer the ribs in a slow cooker, together with the onions, garlic, salt, oregano and chili powder. Pour in the reduced cooking liquid, cover lid and cook on low for about 4 to 5 hours. Remove lid and continue cooking until the sauce has thickened.

5. Remove the beef from the slow cooker and place it on a serving dish, serve with extra sauce on top.

6. Put the ribs, onion, garlic, 2 teaspoons salt, the chili powder and oregano in a

slow cooker. Pour in the wine sauce and cook, covered, on high for 3 1/2 hours. Uncover and cook until the ribs are falling apart, about 45 minutes more. Transfer the ribs and sauce to a serving dish and serve.

Notes

COFFEE HONEY GRILLED PORK CHOPS

Ingredients:

- 1 cup strong brewed coffee, room temperature

- 4 sprigs fresh thyme

- 4 pork chops, 1 inch thick, bone-in

- ½ cup local honey

- 2 tablespoons sherry vinegar

- 1 1/2 tablespoon yellow mustard

- 2 garlic cloves, minced

- salt and coarsely ground black pepper, to taste

- 1/2 teaspoon fresh ginger root, grated

Directions:

1. In a large mixing bowl, whisk together the honey, coffee, garlic, mustard, ginger, thyme, salt and pepper. Whisk thoroughly and add the pork chops, toss

to coat pork chops and transfer into a resealable plastic and chill for at least 2 to 3 hours or overnight.

2. Preheat a gas grill to medium-high. Remove the pork from the fridge. Pour the marinade into a saucepan over medium-high heat and bring to steady boil while stirring. Cook until the sauce has reduced in half, for about 12 to 15 minutes. Remove the thyme and discard.

3. Grill the pork chops for about 3 to 4 minutes per side, or until it reaches an internal temperature of 145°C. Remove from heat and let it rest for 5 minutes, serve with the sauce in a bowl.

Notes

Your eyes are a gift, but more often than not we take them and our sight for granted. Our eyes are busy working tirelessly throughout the day, and you've just got to think about what they get exposed to on a daily basis. TV, cell phones, computers, newspapers, books, and signs to name but a few are some of things we expose our eyes to. Because we use our eyes so much without even realizing it, we're more vulnerable to common eye problems such as distorted vision, poor eyesight, and cataracts. As soon as you begin to develop problems with your eyes, your world can change depending on how severe the problem is. But with the right diet and taking precautions, you can do your part and help preserve your eyes and sight for years to come.

To Clearer Vision!

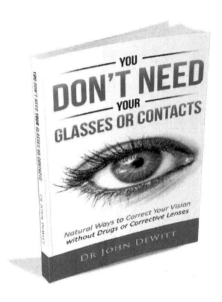

To get my previous book go to amazon.com and please leave a review ☺